SLEEP GREAT

FOR LIFE

The Solution for One of

Life's Greatest Health Risks

Richard J. Nilsen

AllStar
P R E S S

Published by
All Star Press
P.O. Box 2226
Tarpon Springs, FL 34689
www.allstarpress.com

ISBN: 978-1-937376-04-8

Library of Congress Control Number: 2012911251

Cover and jacket designed by All Star Press

Printed in the United States of America

To my beautiful wife, Marta, and my precious baby girl, Natalie. They are the joy of my life and I am so grateful for them.

CONTENTS

INTRODUCTION

Congratulations. Reading this book is about to change your life in a way that you cannot even put a price tag on.

Classic insomnia and the variations of sleep disorders are taking a serious health toll not just on people here in stressed-out America but worldwide. If you are reading this, then chances are that you know full well what I am talking about. You've dealt personally with the impact that lack of sleep can have on your life. Depending on the severity of the problem, it has, no doubt, negatively influenced your life in one form or another.

The bottom line is that, despite what the pharmaceutical companies would have you believe, the truth is that you can't buy a good night's sleep. Many people have attempted to do just that in vain. The prescription-drug market for sleep aids is a billion-dollar industry, yet so many people continue to be plagued by sleep disorders. Drugs can be helpful in the short term, but all too often, they are simply a Band-Aid approach masking the real problem. By the time you finish this guide, you will be well on your way to ditching all prescription drugs for insomnia and overcoming your sleep issues for the remainder of your life. Sound good, right? Believe it, because you have started on the path to eliminating this serious issue in your life and putting it behind you – for good.

One caveat: be patient. We are not going to fix this issue overnight (no pun intended). But I believe that you will overcome your sleep issues, and that aspect of your life will be drastically transformed within the next 28 days. The beautiful thing is that you are going to be able to begin applying the building blocks to a great sleep life starting this very day!

Sleeping great requires, as the old saying goes, having your "ducks in a row." In this book, we are going to lay the proper foundation to get you going in the right direction. Then, we will go over each and every step to overcoming insomnia once and for all. Read this book slowly and soak in all the advice provided.

You will see gradual improvement over the next couple of weeks, and during this process you will expect to succeed and overcome your sleep disorder. You'll know you're almost there the first night that you go to bed with the expectation of having a great night's sleep. When that expectation is followed up by eight or so hours of uninterrupted, great sleep, you'll also know that you are getting closer to permanently kicking this problem.

How can I be so sure? Well, I went through very debilitating insomnia just a few years ago. It started out pretty innocently but snowballed from there. Pretty soon, I was spending all day worrying about what would happen that evening. Would I be able to get to sleep? If it happened again, how would I make it through work the next day? The stress was unbelievable. It led to a deep depression that was hard to mask both at work and in front of friends and family. A domino effect had been created that was wreaking havoc in my life.

My wife couldn't solve the problem. No person could help me. But I found the answers to solving my serious sleep disorder, and I felt it was my responsibility to help as many people as possible by writing this book.

The steps I took to solve my insomnia are all here in this guide. I feel a deep sense of compassion when I hear of someone who is struggling with insomnia. I know full well how serious it can be and what a risk it can present to your overall well-being.

Let's get started.

NOTE: Although many people can personally attest to the effectiveness of the ideas presented in this book, this book is not a substitute for professional medical advice. Always discuss serious medical conditions with your family doctor.

CHAPTER ONE

Impact of the Lack of Sleep

"So many people are sleep deprived. We're living in a time of unprecedented sleep debt."
- Carol Ash, DO, Sleep For Life Center

Insomnia is one of the most serious health risks that a person can face in their lifetime. Everyone goes through at least a period of having trouble sleeping, and often this is caused by some form of difficulty in that person's life. But others deal with this issue on an every-day, on-going basis. It is when insomnia becomes a regular part of life that one has to be very concerned about the subsequent health issues that can follow and the negative impact it can have on the quality of life.

"There is plenty of compelling evidence that sleep is the most important predictor of how long you will live – perhaps more important than whether you smoke, exercise or have high blood pressure or cholesterol levels," explained William Dement, Stanford University psychiatry professor.[1]

Let's see why by looking at all of the different health and life issues that can result from chronic insomnia.

Anxiety

Restlessness

Depression

Difficulty concentrating

Exasperating fears

Decreased work productivity

Lower quality of life

Poor mood and emotional stability

Short temperedness and irritability

Reduced immune system

Risk of physical problems: high blood pressure, diabetes, heart disease, etc.

Lack of energy to exercise

Lack of energy / motivation to perform everyday tasks

Less energy for sex

Altered metabolism, which promotes fat storage

Inflammation and weight gain

Slower reaction time

Impaired metabolism, which can lead to depression

Elevated stress hormones

The ability to handle stress declines exponentially

Developing plaque

That last item may seem strange, but getting one more hour of sleep can reduce calcifications by up to 33 percent.[2] Experts are not sure how or why, but the evidence regarding plaque is rock solid.

A new study has found that individuals who suffer from insomnia have heightened nighttime blood pressure, which can lead to cardiac problems. The research, published in the journal *Sleep*, measured the 24-hour blood pressure levels of insomniacs compared to sound sleepers.

"Whereas blood pressure decreases in regular sleepers and gives their heart a rest, insomnia provokes higher nighttime blood pressure that can cause long-term cardiovascular risks and damage the heart," says leading author Paola A. Lanfranchi, a professor at the University of Montreal.[3]

COMPOUNDING EFFECT

Sleep debt works just like financial debt. Before you realize it, you have a serious problem. You build up sleep debt throughout the week. There are numerous medical studies that prove prolonged lack of sleep can lead to many serious problems including heart disease, high blood pressure, obesity, digestive problems, diabetes, sleep apnea, and even stroke.

"Our alertness level is even more impacted by several days of reduced sleep. If we miss 1-2 hours of sleep over 6-7 consecutive nights, our alertness level drops to dangerously low levels. As many as 15-20% of all transportation accidents are fatigue-related." [4]

This creates a destructive cycle that can be difficult to reverse for many individuals.

SLEEP FACTS

According to the findings of a 2007 study by the United States Department of Health and Human Services, approximately 64 million Americans regularly suffer from insomnia each year, and it is 1.4 times more common in women than men.[5] There is little doubt that this massive number has grown in the past three years.

Fifty-eight percent of adults in the U.S. experience symptoms of insomnia a few nights a week or more.[6]

Forty-four percent of U.S. adults are considered "problem sleepers." About one-fifth of those surveyed used drugs to counter-act insomnia at least once per week, and nearly 24 percent "depended" on sleep medication.[7] *Consumer Reports* magazine found that 38 percent of those who had taken medication in the past month had been doing so for a minimum of two months. Who wants that?

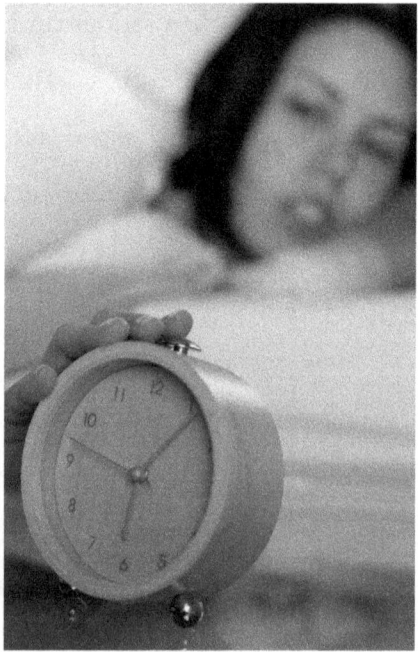

The same leading magazine reported that the most common cause was stress. Respondents worried about issues such as money, health, job security and family.

In 2001, only 38 percent of adults were getting a minimum of eight hours of sleep each night. Within only seven years this percentage had dropped to an alarming 26 percent.[8]

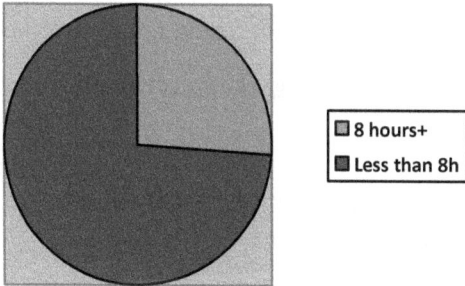

By 2008 just over one out of every four individuals was getting eight hours of sleep each night. That is a shockingly low percentage of people obtaining the amount of sleep they need each night to function at their best the next day. Now granted, some people can get by just fine on less sleep, but too many people are not getting the "shut eye" that they require to function at their best.

"Reactions, memory capacity, everything slows down really fast – already after the first night [of insomnia]. Today we know of 88 kinds of sleep disorders. For 50 percent of patients, the disturbance is mental," explained Thomas Penzel of the Charite Hospital in Berlin, Germany.

Consider that statement. Half of all sleep disorder patients can attribute their disturbance to a mental issue. I believe that is a very conservative number, especially if you eliminate the people with proven physical issues such as sleep apnea. If anything, the percentage is much higher.

According to the U.S. National Transportation Safety Board, the leading cause of fatal-to-the-driver heavy truck crashes is fatigue-related. Fatigue and sleep deprivation accounted for 31-percent of the cases; whereas, alcohol and other drug use accounted for 29 percent.[9]

Sleep deprivation was believed to be a major factor in several high-profile incidents such as the Exxon Valdez oil spill (which killed no telling how much wildlife), the Chernobyl nuclear accident, the Three Mile Island nuclear accident, and even the space shuttle Challenger.

Just how many people are affected by sleep issues? A survey in February 2009 by the National Association of Home Builders, which included builders and architects, predicted that over 60 percent of custom-made houses would have dual master bedrooms by the year 2015.[10]

People are trying to "get away" and find a solution to their sleep disorders, even if it means sleeping apart from their significant other.

THE ULTIMATE HEALTH CONSEQUENCE

Oh, and I forgot one item from the list that started this chapter. In a very small percentage of cases, when a sleep disorder gets to a critical stage, it can lead to the ultimate health consequence. Notable high-profile deaths which we have seen recently in the news include actor Heath Ledger and superstar Michael Jackson. Both big name stars were tormented by sleep disorders and died from taking an overdose of insomnia-related medicines.

How horrible it is to see what happened in both of these cases. Here were two of the most talented individuals of our generation and both died such sad deaths. Based on reliable reports, insomnia was the root cause that led to their very poor decisions.

Thankfully, we're not going to have to worry about any of these issues detailed in this chapter, because this book is presenting to you the foundation for eliminating your sleep disorder – permanently.

QUESTIONS:

Do I currently suffer from sleep debt?

How many hours per night of consecutive sleep have I averaged over the past week?

CHAPTER TWO

Causes of Sleep Disorders

"We live in a time when we are working harder, eating unhealthier diets, exercising less, taking more prescription drugs, and sleeping less than at any other point in history."

– Lena Edwards, MD[1]

There are a variety of factors in one's life that can lead to a sleep disorder. Most commonly, some form of stress has reached a breaking point. Your ability to adapt to the stress has failed, and now you are unable to rest peacefully at night. The result can be a debilitating problem.

The work environment is one of the leading causes of stress in one's life. From project deadlines set by supervisors who don't understand everything involved, to personality clashes with other employees, the work environment is fertile ground for stress.

Life issues that can lead to a sleep disorder include:

Fear

Anxiety

Personal issues

Significant change in one's life

Financial stress

Work-related stress

Lack of detachment from work

Poor job satisfaction

Lack of control

Lack of detachment from technology

Poor sleep hygiene (see Chapter Four)

Physical pain

Grief

Illness

Lack of faith

Guilt or shame for sinful or immoral behavior

Winter blues/Seasonal depression

WARNING SIGNS OF AN INCREASED STRESS LEVEL

One of the common behavioral reactions to stress can be an exaggeration of an existing habit. Maybe one of your responses is overeating, and you suddenly notice yourself eating way more than you usually do. Or it could be cigarettes, and you suddenly find yourself smoking more frequently.

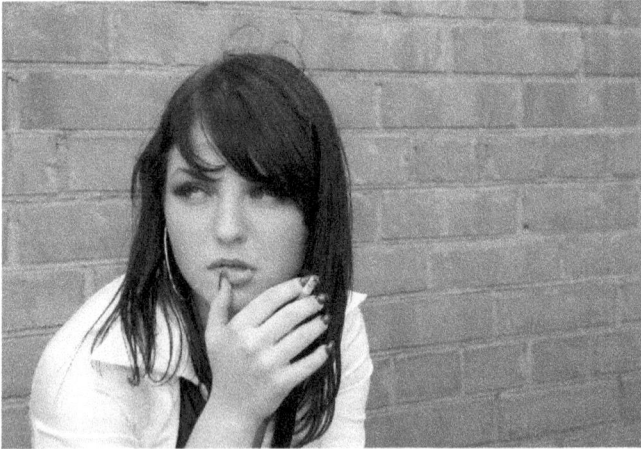

These will be important factors to keep a close eye on after you solve your sleep disorder. Insomnia can come back, but only if you let it. Be confident that you won't let that happen because you will have established a solid foundation. Your precious sleep life will not be built on shifting sands.

The following are some red flags to watch out for. Feel free to add to this list based on your own experience:

Muscular tension and physical pain

Obsessive thoughts

Closing yourself off from others

Increased levels of bad habits – e.g. smoking, overeating, etc.

Tics and small muscle spasms – face, eyes, etc.

Sweating

Fatigue

Increased need to urinate – often a sign of depression

Ulcers

Difficulty concentrating

Feeling overwhelmed with your workload

Feeling overwhelmed with responsibilities

Mood swings

Lack of motivation

Other [list your own] _____

QUESTIONS:

Now, it is time to honestly ask yourself: What is it in my life that is contributing to or even directly causing my insomnia? What in my life could I change tomorrow that would help eliminate this issue in the long run?

When did this problem start?

How did it get worse?

What do I feel are the top three causes of my insomnia?

_____

_____

_____

The more honest you can be with yourself, the better your chance of diagnosing the root causes. It may be one main culprit or a combination of negative factors. Remember: forewarned is forearmed. Be prepared and don't let yourself get blindsided again.

CHAPTER THREE

Benefits of Great Sleep

"The best bridge between despair and hope is a good night's sleep."
– E. Joseph Cossman, Entrepreneur & Author

Now that we have talked about the negatives of insomnia and sleep disorders, let's talk about some positive things. After all, *Sleep Great for Life* is about the wonderful experience that sleep will be in your life on a long-term and permanent basis.

Sleeping great has so many benefits that they can't all be quantified. When we sleep well, we often take those benefits for granted. It's when we don't sleep well that we realize how important sleep is to our overall health, mindset and well-being.

The benefits of great sleep include:

Feeling rested

Feeling energetic

The immune system is strengthened during sleep

The body makes repairs and tissues are regenerated during sleep

More energy = better sex life

Lower risk of injury

Better looking skin

Sharper thought process during the day

More energy = more productive

Maintain proper weight

Better overall mood

Better communication

and the list goes on.

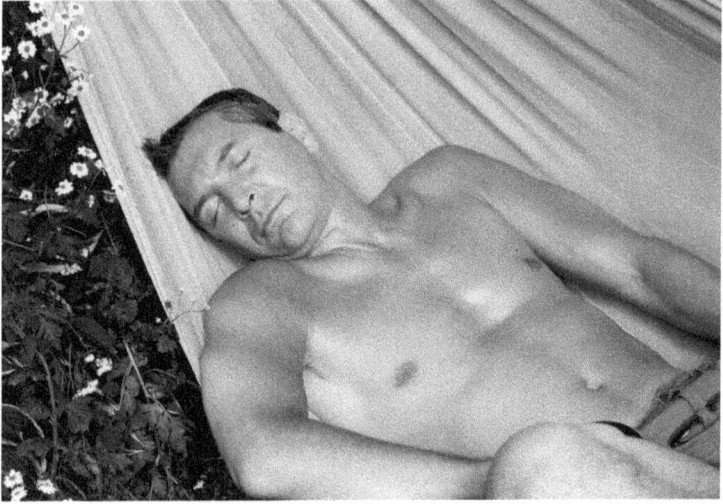

Shouldn't great sleep look like this? All the women reading the book are nodding emphatically.

Now we start getting to the good stuff. In the next chapter you will learn how to lay the right foundation for nights of great sleep. This isn't rocket science. Yet, it's amazing how many people fail to apply proper sleep hygiene. I know - I was one of them.

CHAPTER FOUR

Sleep Hygiene - Laying the Foundation for a Great Night's Sleep

"The physiological mechanisms involved are complex, but in a nutshell, bad sleep hygiene disrupts normal hormonal patterns that need to be reset at night. Insulin, growth hormone, melatonin and thyroid hormone can be affected negatively by poor sleep."

\- Bryant Stamford, The Body Shop[1]

A house built on shifting sands…well, you know the famous verse. We need a solid sleep foundation, and this chapter will go over each and every step that you need to incorporate into your life as soon as possible.

Sleep hygiene describes good habits that can help give you the best chance at refreshing, rejuvenating sleep. There are several basic tenets of sleep hygiene, which include:

Go to bed at the same time each night.

Get up at the same time each morning.

Spend at least part of each day outdoors in natural light.

Use your bed only for sleep and sex.

Don't drink or ingest anything with caffeine in the evening.

Don't share your bedroom with children or pets.

Just as sleep hygiene describes the good habits you need, many sleep issues are the result of the bad habits we develop over the course of a long period of time.

Sleep Great for Life offers several other sleep hygiene suggestions, all of which I can personally attest were helpful to me in licking insomnia. Let's dive right into each of these so that you can begin applying them immediately in your life.

AVOID LIQUIDS AND CAFFEINE

Let's start with the basics. You want to avoid all liquids a minimum of two hours prior to bedtime. And I don't just mean alcohol. That's a given, but we will address that more later.

The last thing you want to happen, when you're trying to put an end to your sleep disorder, is unnecessary "getting up" in the middle of the night.

This is common sense, along with avoiding any type of caffeine. Remember that caffeine is not just found in tea and coffee; it is also found in food items such as candy, especially chocolate, although to a much lesser extent. Some over-the-counter cold and headache remedies are high in caffeine, so check with your pharmacist if you are using items such as these.

AVOID HEAVY MEALS

You definitely want to avoid eating or drinking anything close to bedtime that could disturb your sleep. Eating a big meal within two hours of bedtime is simply not good for your health and not good for your sleep hygiene. Nor do you want your stomach to be growling while you're lying in bed. So, clearly we want to be somewhere in the middle and that is not difficult to accomplish on a daily basis as long as one just eats dinner at a regular hour and keeps snacks to a minimum. Your body weight, cholesterol, and overall health will thank you for it.

LIMIT NAPPING

Resist napping if you can. At the most keep it to a 10- or 15-minute power nap earlier in the day. Anything more than that runs the risk of disrupting your sleep that evening.

MOVE THAT CLOCK

One of the problems I quickly identified during my insomnia was seeing the clock throughout the night. I would have to get up, usually due to my severe restlessness. Consequently, I couldn't avoid seeing the big LCD display on my clock.

"1:15 a.m.! Are you kidding me?" I would say to myself, lying there in the dark, extremely frustrated. "I've only been asleep two hours, and now I'm wide awake and not going back to sleep. This can't be happening again."

This was a regular routine for me, and it was seriously impacting any chance I had to relax and get back to sleep.

Of course, I still needed a clock. I had to get up for work – at some point in the morning – and get ready for the day. Accomplishing that task each morning was a tremendous struggle during my bout with insomnia.

The solution was to move the clock 90 degrees and out of plain sight. I did the same for my wife's clock, which had been positioned just so that depending on where her head was, I might accidentally see her clock. Her clock had to be re-positioned as well. It was a simple change but it helped me tremendously.

ASSESS YOUR ENVIRONMENT

Are you comfortable in your current sleep environment? What can you do to improve the situation? How is your mattress? Is your pillow a good fit? Ask yourself all the relevant questions.

For starters, you want everything to be extremely comfortable. The temperature of the room is critical. Make

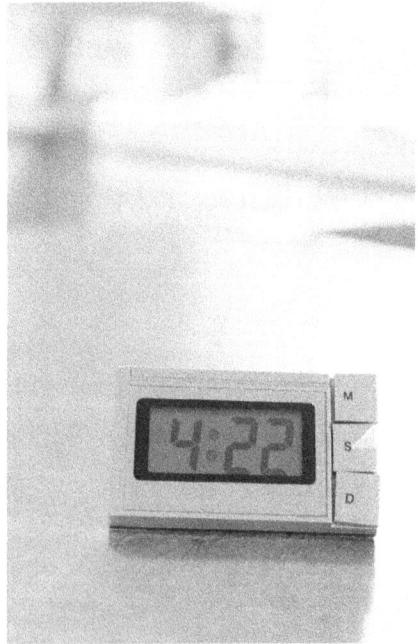

sure the room is dark and the temperature just right for you. Most people prefer a room that is more on the cool end. You may be different, but at this stage of your life, you surely know what the right temperature is.

I like a room that is slightly cooler than the other rooms in the home, and I also prefer to have a ceiling fan running during the night to keep the air flowing. I used to employ another fan that served as "white noise" because I liked the humming sound which would block out other noises. I have long since gotten away from relying on that fan.

Sleep masks, earplugs, and blackout curtains are among the tools that people can rely on to make their bedrooms compatible with their sleep preferences.

Now make sure your bed is comfortable. Ideally, you are spending one-third of your entire day on that mattress and pillow. Despite that, few people put much research or time into finding the right mattress and pillow for them. If you have ever slept in a hotel or someone else's house, then you know very well that there are great variations in these items. Make sure yours are the best you can afford.

A mattress pad is one great way to make your bed much more comfy without spending a fortune. Wal-Mart, for example, sells mattress pads that mimic down feathers for a fraction of the cost found at high-end stores.

How about noise and lighting? Make sure the room is dark enough and that there are no noises in the room that are disturbing to you during the night.

If you have a spouse or loved one, ask yourself if that person is an issue? Many a snorer, for example, has ruined someone else's sleep. At least during this recovery stage, you may have to sleep alone if the other person does present a deterrent. After you've licked this insomnia, you can likely return to your original sleep arrangements.

EXERCISE

Try to get into a routine of exercising each day. It is doubly good if you can do it outside during the day, where you will be able to get some sunlight and, consequently, some Vitamin D. Even if the weather is bad, you can still get your cardiovascular activity in by exercising at home. Find some space in your house, purchase a DVD of an aerobics class, and accomplish your cardiovascular exercise on a daily basis.

Other forms of exercise that can be done in the house include yoga, jumping rope, and jogging or walking on a treadmill, etc.

Make sure not to exercise too close to bedtime. You don't want your body stimulated in the hours when you should be shutting down for the night. That's a recipe for nighttime trouble.

EAT WELL

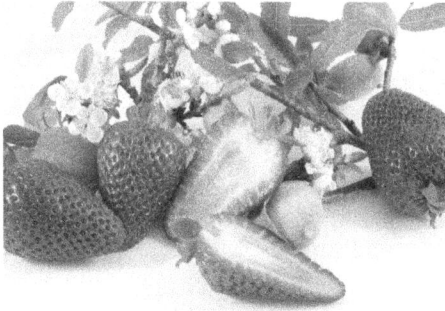

In addition to avoiding heavy meals and liquids close to bedtime, it just makes common sense that you should immediately get into a daily routine of eating well. By keeping a good diet, you will maintain a more ideal weight and just feel better overall.

Avoid evening meals that are high in fat. Also, avoid any foods that are likely to cause you heartburn or indigestion. The effects of spicy food, for example, worsen as you lie down. Avoid foods high in protein. Foods rich in protein contain an amino acid known as tyrosine. Tyrosine is believed to stimulate brain activity, the last thing you need late in the evening.

As for foods that are believed to aid the sleep process, look towards milk (and other items containing calcium), honey, and bananas.

USE TECHNOLOGY TO YOUR ADVANTAGE

Don't want to miss that favorite television show that starts at 10:00 p.m.? Well, that is what DVRs and VCRs are for. DVRs are wonderful in that you can set up a regular, scheduled taping every time your favorite show airs. You can also easily record the remainder of a show if you find yourself getting sleepy. Use modern technology to your advantage. Your sleep is too important.

WRITE DOWN YOUR THOUGHTS

I am a firm believer that by putting your thoughts, especially regarding problems, to paper, you can release them from your mind. Then, you can wake up the next day and, at that time, address the issue(s) when you can actually do something about it. Another benefit of doing this is that you will not lose that great idea that you just had while lying in bed!

Make sure you do not go to bed with your mind racing or with problems still pending. Put them "to bed" for the night, and then you will be able to put yourself to bed – peacefully.

PUT GOALS IN PERSPECTIVE

What are your main goals in life? Psychologists Richard Ryan and Tim Kasser performed a series of studies a few years back that drew the conclusion that people who made the pursuit of money and materialism a top goal in life had lower well-being. The studies found that these individuals had a variety of personal problems such as higher anxiety and depressive symptoms.[2]

If you are not happy in your life, make sure you are setting the right goals. If the main pursuits in life have no real meaning, then you'll never be satisfied. Consequently, you will worry more, and that can seriously affect your sleep.

Assess your priorities and make the needed adjustments.

EVALUATE YOUR MENTAL STATE

If you suffer from any form of depression, you may not sleep well, at least not on a regular basis. If you believe you have clinical depression or an anxiety disorder, seek your physician's advice immediately. If for some reason you do not have a general practitioner, ask around. Inquire with people you know and trust and ask them if there is a doctor they recommend. It does not have to be a doctor who specializes in this field, as many doctors can recognize and treat depression. One way or another, seek help and do it pronto!

STOP OBSESSING

Lots of us obsess about various things in our lives. Obsessive thoughts can negatively impact our sleep. If we are an obsessive personality, it is important to turn this trait into a positive.

"I will sleep great tonight." If you need to obsess with any type of thought, make it this one. Repeat this to yourself throughout the day if any negative thought enters your mind. Then, when you are lying in bed, repeat this statement three times...and believe it!

We will come back to this valuable phrase more in chapter eight.

AVOID STIMULATION

Many people may not realize that this includes the Internet. Don't be surfing the web shortly before bedtime. In my opinion this is much worse than television, which many experts commonly mention as a contributing cause of insomnia.

The light from the computer screen can certainly mess with your body's internal clock, much more so than a television parked 10 feet or further away.

Don't be checking your work email one final time before bed, either. I know I have been guilty of that on too many occasions. There is nothing that can't wait until the morning. Just think: if it is a problem, do you really want to handle it at this late hour, or if you can't, do you want to go to bed having to worry about it? It's a lose-lose situation. Avoid it.

It can be difficult at first to make this disconnect from technology, but it is well worth it.

MITIGATE STRESS

Sit down and spend some time analyzing what exactly is causing stress in your life. Are there things that are regularly causing stress which you have control over? When you really analyze the situations, you will be surprised to find how many issues you actually do have control over. In other words, you can make changes to eliminate or reduce the stress that is brought on by these issues.

In my particular situation a few years ago, my wife and I were running a small business on the side. I was managing the emails and orders that would come in and was basically serving as a customer service representative. Many times, I would deal with this immediately after a long day at my regular, full-time job or shortly before bedtime. Other times, I would ignore the business for a day or two and then try to play catch up. Neither situation was good. And both choices were creating unnecessary stress in my life. I told my wife that we would have to shut down the business because it simply wasn't a healthy thing for me. We eventually found a better solution and were able to keep the side business going, but most importantly, I got that stress removed from my busy lifestyle. This didn't cure my insomnia, but it certainly alleviated a burden and helped me recover more quickly.

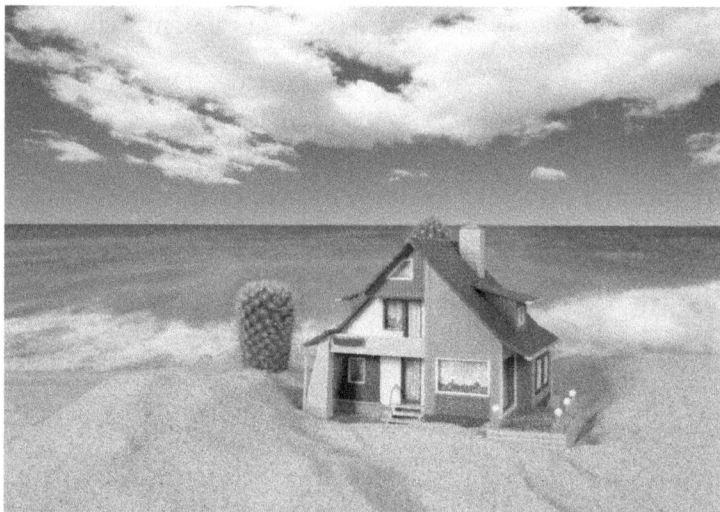

Make sure your sleep is built on a solid foundation.

FIND A GOOD READ

You want to go to bed with the right frame of mind. Your mental state is critical to your success. I highly recommend finding a good book or two to read, and find one that is an inspirational work. There are many great self-help books from Tony Robbins, the late Norman Vincent Peale, and others. If that type of stuff doesn't keep you interested, then specifically find a book that has a positive message. You do not want a book that presents any type of suspense. Save that for when your sleep disorder is ancient history. Besides, it won't be long!

SUMMARY

I know this was quite a bit to take in, especially in one reading. Begin making changes immediately. You likely will not get it all right in one day, so go back and read this chapter on sleep hygiene so that you don't overlook anything. Keep notes for yourself, if necessary, and make sure you get on the path to a solid sleep hygiene foundation as soon as possible.

QUESTIONS:

Which sleep hygiene items am I failing at right now? Note all areas where you can make improvements.

REVIEW:

Right now, mark one week ahead on your calendar, mobile device, or whatever you use for scheduling items. After the one week deadline arrives and ask yourself: Am I fully committed to each of the sleep hygiene items presented in this chapter? If not, then start again.

CHAPTER FIVE

Consult Your Physician

"Studies have demonstrated that poor sleep and susceptibility to colds go hand in hand, and scientists think it could be a reflection of the role sleep plays in maintaining the body's defenses. . . . Sleep and immunity, it seems, are tightly linked."

– Anahad O'Connor[1]

I believe there is a wealth of great information in this book that can help so many people with different forms of sleep disorders. However, with that said, there are many cases of insomnia that are directly related to a medical condition. Several health issues can negatively affect one's sleep. Just to name a few:

Back and neck pain
Chronic pain

Sciatica

Incontinence

Drugs and withdrawing from medicine

Until recently, there was no defined medical field devoted to the study of insomnia. Now sleep medicine is a recognized subspecialty within several medical fields here in the United States including internal medicine, pediatrics, psychiatry, and neurology.

Sleep apnea is one of the most commonly known and widely publicized medical reasons that explain why someone can be suffering from poor sleep. Individuals with sleep apnea don't realize that they are not experiencing the five stages of sleep and, consequently, they are tired throughout the day because they did not experience the restorative power of a great night's sleep.

Another condition that has been seen in numerous advertisements is RLS, or restless leg syndrome.

You don't hear much about narcolepsy anymore, but this condition, which is characterized by excessive sleepiness during the day, affects about one in every 2,000 people.[2]

This book is not for these types of issues, although I do feel the concepts presented here can help many individuals who are not sleeping well due to pain-related issues.

CHAPTER SIX

Sleep Medicines and Supplements

"All sedative drugs have the potential of causing psychological dependence where the individual cannot psychologically accept that they can sleep without the drugs."

– Wikipedia.org

There are a lot of potential side effects with pretty much every prescription sleep medicine. I will not go into all of them here, but if you have any in your possession, simply read the warning labels. There is a reason those warnings are on the label, and it is not at the willingness of the pharmaceutical companies. In most cases, they have been forced to put those warnings on their products.

Sleep-driving made headlines in the spring of 2006 when Rep. Patrick Kennedy crashed his car after taking Ambien along with a sedative known as Phenergan. Ambien is one of the most popular sleep aids on the market.

As the world saw in the cases of Heath Ledger, Michael Jackson, and most recently, Whitney Houston, the use of sleep medication can lead to more serious doses or concoctions. Why would these individuals have taken such crazy risks? Because the basic sleep medications stopped working. The root cause of the sleep disorder was never solved.

"The bottom line is that these pills [sleep medicine] are dangerous," stated Dr. Isadore Rosenfeld, author of *Doctor of the Heart.*[1]

Don't get me wrong. These medicines serve an important purpose. I have taken many a sleeping pill over the years, including Ambien, and was thankful for it. However, I also learned the hard way that when one's sleep disorder is serious enough, sleeping pills do not work. Sleeping pills are also designed to be a short-term solution. Thanks to the solid principles presented here in this book, I have not taken a single sleeping pill in years.

There are some over-the-counter supplements that many people believe help with insomnia. Before taking any supplement, be sure to check with your doctor.

POPULAR HERBAL SUPPLEMENTS

Melatonin is believed to be able to help insomnia without altering the individual's sleep pattern, unlike many prescription drugs. It is not addictive, though the risks of using melatonin are not fully known.

Valerian, like melatonin, falls under the Dietary Supplement Health and Education Act of 1994, which allows "medicines" such as this one to bypass the oversight of the Food and Drug Administration (FDA). Derived from the roots of the valerian plant, this herbal medicine is used for a variety of purposes, one of which is treating sleep disorders. Some people find it to work well, especially when used over a period of time. As with melatonin, the risks of using valerian are not fully known.

Many experts believe both of these products are fairly harmless and do help many individuals with anxiety and sleep disorders. However, there are several adverse side effects that Valerian has been known to cause in some people. Valerian is also not to be used at the same time as other depressants, such as alcohol. If you are using herbal supplements, make sure you do the research and understand the risks involved.

Remember **kava-kava**? This popular anti-anxiety herbal pill was pulled from store shelves a few years ago when there was a proven link found between kava and liver damage. Kava was also found to have documented adverse interactions with several prescription and non-prescription drugs. Kava is an excellent example of why we want to weed ourselves off of all types of unnecessary, unregulated supplements. With no FDA oversight, we simply don't know the possible risks.

VITAMINS/NATURAL REMEDIES

Magnesium is known to relax the muscles. You can improve your diet and increase your magnesium intake without a supplement. Foods with magnesium include almonds, brown rice, swiss chard, spinach, and lima beans.

The **amino acid tryptophan** is found in certain foods. It is used by the brain to create the hormone we all know and love as serotonin.

"The key to getting enough tryptophan to your brain to sleep well at night is to combine a tryptophan-rich food with a carbohydrate-rich food," explained Chet Day on his *Health And Beyond* website. "This is because ingesting a carbohydrate-rich food causes your body to release insulin, which diverts many of your other amino acids away from your brain, leaving tryptophan with little competition to cross your blood-brain barrier to gain access to your brain."

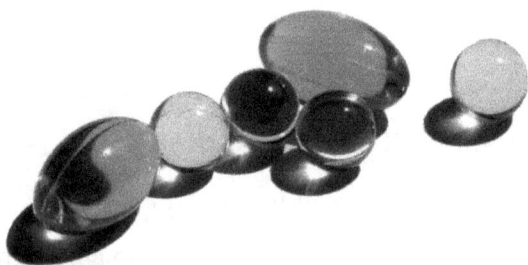

Foods rich in the amino acid tryptophan include whole grains, soy milk, sunflower and sesame seeds, and nuts such as hazelnuts and peanuts.

OUR GOAL

Every person who reads *Sleep Great for Life* will, hopefully, wean themselves off of all sleep medicines and unregulated supplements and solve the problem naturally. I believe in my heart that by setting the proper foundation and following the steps detailed in this book, that you will do just that.

CHAPTER SEVEN

The Five Stages of Sleep

"The growing seduction of the Internet, video games and endless TV channels? Never disconnecting from work? No matter how it happened, millions of chronically sleep-deprived Americans are putting their health, quality of life, and even <u>length</u> of life in jeopardy."
– Lori Miller Kase[1]

Although understanding sleep is not necessary in order to conquer insomnia, it does help to understand how the sleep process works. There are five stages of sleep that help restore our bodies.

Stage One is the transitional stage when everything begins to slow down, from your brain waves to muscle activity.

Stage Two begins light sleep where heart and brain activity slows and body temperature drops.

Stage Three begins the deep sleep stages. Known as delta sleep, Stages Three and Four are when your body restoration and repair take place. If you are awakened suddenly during either of these stages, you will feel extremely groggy and uncomfortable. This is why it is so important NOT to take long naps. If you reach deep sleep in a nap, you're in trouble. If you are awakened, you will feel like crap, in plain English, and it will take some time to wake back up. If you sleep too long during the nap, your body isn't going to be in a big rush for the real sleep later than evening.

Stage Five is REM sleep, which is characterized by rapid and shallow breathing, rapid eye movements, and also fast brain waves.

These sleep stages are repeated several times during the night. Your body needs to go through these stages to replenish itself and experience all the great benefits of a wonderful night's sleep.

Now let's get to work, so we can begin to enjoy these five stages each and every night…for the rest of your life!

CHAPTER EIGHT

Step-by-Step Solution: Sleep Great for Life!

"I will sleep great tonight."

– [insert your own name here]

It's time to get into the heart and soul of *Sleep Great for Life*. This is where the work we have done up until this point is going to pay off in leaps and bounds.

STEP ONE

Before we begin, we need to make sure we have laid the proper foundation through superior sleep hygiene. Even if you have not perfected all of these steps, keep working on each and every item presented in Chapter Four. It is critical that you are doing everything you can to create the best possible environment for great sleep. Follow the procedures discussed in the sleep hygiene chapter to the letter of the law.

Continue to work on these factors and make them a regular part of your life until you can honestly give yourself an A grade for sleep hygiene. For every section that you fail, knock off a letter grade.

<u>To summarize these points:</u>

Avoid all liquids a minimum of two hours prior to bedtime.

Avoid eating a big meal within two hours of bedtime.

Do not nap more than 15 minutes during the course of the day; sleeping is for nighttime.

Move your clock out of view.

Make sure your sleep environment is comfortable – temperature, mattress, etc.

Use the bedroom only for sleeping and sex.

Get into a routine of exercising each day.

Eat well and improve your diet.

Write your problems down. Don't let them fester.

Create non-monetary goals for your life.

Evaluate your mental state. Are there any issues that need to be addressed?

Stop obsessing negatively. Confidently repeat "I will sleep great tonight" throughout the day.

Do not surf the web close to bedtime. Shut down all electronics well before that time.

Read a good (non-suspenseful) book before going to bed.

I can't emphasize enough how important sleep hygiene is to this entire process. Not completing these steps would be like a professional athlete never practicing. Come game time, what type of foundation would that player have?

While you are perfecting your sleep hygiene, you can begin the key steps that are the solution for eliminating insomnia. This is the critical starting point for *Sleep Great for Life*. Let's begin now to train your mind to expect a great night's sleep. It will happen. Expect it.

STEP TWO

Yes, we are going to change our thought pattern. I have my wonderful sister Kathy to thank for making me cognizant of an important fact about our family. In discussing my insomnia issues with her, she explained to me that there exists an "obsessive trait" within our family. Although I never considered myself an addictive personality, I realized that she was right.

It was true that I had been obsessing over this problem in my life. It had gotten so bad that I had absolutely no confidence that I would be able to get any rest when I put myself to bed for the evening. I worried constantly throughout the day over the dreaded bedtime that would come later in the evening. The stress heightened with every hour closer to bedtime. This created a domino effect. The more sleepless nights I suffered, the more I worried throughout the day and the more sleepless nights I had. It was a vicious cycle.

Insomnia is not something I would wish on my worst enemy. It is a crushing feeling to go to bed, desperately needing a good night's sleep, and getting just the opposite. Then, you struggle to get out of bed in the morning to get ready for an 8-hour-plus workday. It became a pure hell.

My sleep disorder had reached a zenith – something had to change drastically. How did I begin on a new path? I reversed the thought process. If my negative obsessing could get me into this jam, then repeating positive thoughts throughout the day could help me climb out of this hole.

I started telling myself during the course of the day "I will sleep great tonight." Whenever a negative thought entered my mind, I would immediately try to replace it with positive affirmations. I had to be disciplined in doing this, while at the same time convincing myself that I believed what I was saying. The process was challenging but very do-able.

YOUR MINDSET

Whether you realize it or not, you have a negative mindset – at least when it comes to your sleeping habits. You probably don't have confidence that you are going to get a great night's sleep. Why would you? Sleep, or lack thereof, has been a major source of stress in your life recently. However, we are going to change that. You are going to re-train your brain. This is at the core of our philosophy.

The great American philosopher Ralph Waldo Emerson stated, **"A man is what he thinks about all day long."** How true this is.

We want to ingrain positive thoughts in our mindset. We have a step-by-step process for accomplishing that, and, consequently, altering our thought process from a negative mindset to one that anticipates and expects positive results.

The first thing we need to do is to eliminate unnecessary worries. This begins with worrying about our insomnia. Admittedly or not, if you are suffering from insomnia, then going to bed is not a pleasant experience. If it is not an experience you are looking forward to, and it is something you "have to do" eventually each day, then you are going to fret about it. You may not fret about it all day long, like I did at the peak of my sleep disorder, but you are going to worry about the dreaded bedtime. And that form of worry impedes your sleep.

In so many situations in life, worrying accomplishes nothing. What you do often accomplish when you worry is that you reduce the level of enjoyment in your life. And who wants that? Start right now by replacing negative thoughts with positive affirmations.

Create a list of favorable phrases, such as "I will sleep great tonight," "Sleep is great," and "I love sleep." Engrain these thoughts in your mind. If a negative worry or thought pops up, immediately replace that thought with one of your key phrases. Do this religiously over the next several weeks. Pretty soon, thinking positively about sleep will become second nature. As you start to have some good nights of sleep, you will begin to reaffirm these positive thoughts with statements such as "I slept great last night. That felt so good."

STEP THREE

One of the absolutely key factors in overcoming insomnia is to relax. But, of course, that is easier said than done. During the worst stages of my sleep disorder, my nerves were completely on edge mainly because I was stressed at work and even more stressed out about getting a good night's sleep. This created a domino effect and made my insomnia a major problem. It was one of the two biggest stumbling blocks that I experienced preventing me from overcoming my insomnia.

There are some ways to overcome this difficulty and get your entire body to relax. First, you must recognize that you have to relax. There is no other option, because the alternative results in insomnia. Simply put, you cannot get a restful night's sleep if your nerves are fried.

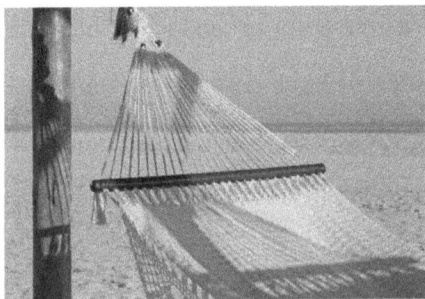

You will repeat the following words when you find yourself restless in bed. The two keyword phrases to submerge into your subconscious are **"Relax"** and **"Deep Sleep."** Why? Because those are the exact two things you are asking your body to do. Consequently, you are ordering your body to do just that. Just as your body responds to negative thought processes, I believe it also responds to orders.

Begin by repeating the following phrases:

"Relax." Calmly take a deep breath. Exhale.

"Relax." Slowly and deliberately, remain calm.

"Deep sleep."

"Relax." Calmly take a deep breath. Exhale.

"Relax." Slowly and deliberately, remain calm.

"Deep sleep."

Now repeat the above simple process and do it with more and more confidence. Focus on the words, as they are detailed instructions to your whole body.

As you lie in bed, you can also repeat other key phrases:

"Calm."

"Tranquility."

"Peace."

"Love."

"Blessings."

"God's Love."

"Gratitude."

By focusing on these positive affirmations and stating them out loud, you are training your mind and body to relax and, consequently, experience great sleep.

DE-STRESS

Being relaxed throughout the day will aid you come nighttime. Obviously, the first and most important step is to remove as much stress as possible from your lifestyle. Remember that you can say "no" to more things than you think. As you learn to say "no," you'll find yourself with less stress and more time to relax.

Another common relaxation method is meditation. Meditation is not something that you do once or twice a day. It requires daily discipline. Mornings are often the best to find quiet time and perform meditation. To learn more about meditation techniques, do some searches online or check out a book at your local library.

TEST YOUR BREATHING

A vital part of the relaxation process is proper breathing. Even though we breathe throughout the day without even thinking about it, this process can be negatively affected by stress, especially the type of stress that can result in a sleeping disorder.

There is a standard test to determine if you are breathing properly. When you first lie down in bed, place one hand on your chest and your other hand on your belly. Distract yourself by focusing on something other than this process. After a minute or two, take notice of which of your hands is being pushed up when you breathe in.

You are not getting the proper oxygen into your body if only the hand on your chest is being raised.

Ideally, you want both hands, one after the other, to rise and fall as you breathe. If this is not happening, then chances are that you are not fully relaxed. Otherwise, you would be breathing properly, and your body and all of its many organs would benefit appropriately.

TIP: FOCUS ON THE BLACK

What do you see when you are lying in the dark trying to go to sleep? It should be nothing. It should be all black. You can focus on what you see and that may just distract you from what is running through your mind at the moment. I began to tell myself "focus on the black." This seemed to be a useful tool to distract myself and increase my chances of falling asleep within a short period of time. For me, it worked a lot better than something like counting sheep.

Focus on the black. It's simple and effective.

STEP FOUR

You are going to start sleeping well because you have followed the first three steps. Acknowledge every night that you have experienced a good night's sleep and be thankful. Say to yourself when you awake, "That was a solid night's sleep. Thank you, Lord." It is very important to reinforce every good experience related to your recovery. The body will build on those positive experiences in much the same way it built on the negative experiences that created your sleep disorder.

CASE STUDY

The key elements of this process were given to an 82-year-old man who was suffering from terrible insomnia. He was ailing with multiple physical conditions, including COPD (Chronic Obstructive Pulmonary Disease), a serious medical condition that affects one's breathing. As a result, he was only getting one to two hours of sleep each night. This had gone on for months, and it was taking a toll on his mental well being.

The first day he applied the elements presented in this book, the man slept for seven hours. The success was repeated for the next several days with consistency.

He focused on the short phrase "deep sleep" as he lay down to bed, and the instant results he experienced were amazing.

The *Sleep Great for Life* formula can work for you.

GREAT SLEEP WITHIN 7 WEEKS

Let's summarize how we are going to overcome our sleep disorder in the next few weeks. We've laid the proper foundation by applying sleep hygiene in our lives. We will constantly evaluate ourselves and make sure we are adhering to all of the sleep hygiene tactics discussed in this book.

Next, we are going to change our thought pattern. We will not let negative thoughts ruin our chances for a great night's sleep. We are going to constantly repeat the positive affirmations throughout the day and at bedtime. No negative thoughts will be allowed. If they do try to creep into our consciousness, we are going to immediately replace them with the various positive thoughts and sayings that we have memorized.

We will de-stress and make sure that we are relaxed when we go to bed. If you are not relaxed and breathing properly, you will not get the restorative sleep you need. It's that simple. Let go of the problems you experienced during the day. Let go of the crappy boss you have or the poor work environment. Recall the "Serenity Prayer" which goes as follows:

God grant me the serenity to accept the things I cannot change;

the courage to change the things I can;

and the wisdom to know the difference.

Living one day at a time;

Enjoying one moment at a time;

Accepting hardships as the pathway to peace;

Taking, as He did, this sinful world as it is, not as I would have it;

Trusting that He will make all things right if I surrender to His will;

That I may be reasonably happy in this life and supremely happy with Him

Forever in the next.

Amen.

Let go of the things that are out of your control.

We are going to be thankful every time that we get a solid night's sleep. We will acknowledge to ourselves that we had a good night's sleep and be thankful for it. By doing this, we are maintaining a positive thought process. Sleep is going to do a 180 and become a positive aspect of your life. Sleep will no longer be a thorn in your side. It will be restorative hours that your mind and body need each day.

All of these steps fit together like pieces of a puzzle. Without one of these steps, we have a very difficult time experiencing great sleep. Instead, we are going to obtain great sleep for life by following the procedure outlined in this book.

It takes commitment. It takes discipline. Sleep is one of the most important aspects of your life. Without it, our health and quality of life suffers greatly.

I purposefully didn't write a 300-page book. It wasn't necessary, and the length of this book allows you to go back and read it multiple times. Everything we have discussed is a stepping stone for great sleep, so let it sink in to your subconscious.

One more chapter: one final step that you may wish to incorporate into your Sleep Great plans.

CHAPTER NINE

Tapping Into a Higher Power

"The Lord is the strength of my life. In this I will have confidence."

– Psalms 27:1

Imagine you were playing a round of golf with your friends and you could have Tiger Woods or Phil Mickelson as your partner. It was your best score against their score. How confident would you be? Or, maybe you're playing tennis doubles, and your teammate is Roger Federer or Rafael Nadal. It is highly likely that you would be as confident as you've ever been about anything in your life. Your weaknesses wouldn't matter. Your partner would come to the rescue and bail you out. Winning would be guaranteed.

You can have that type of partner in the more important game of life when you rely on a higher power instead of your own knowledge and ability. To say God is omnipotent does not even convey the enormity of His power. Think about the Earth. It is just a small part of the universe that we "know." Right now scientists are discovering galaxies that we didn't even know existed a year ago.

Why not put this unbelievable source of strength and power to work for you? Ask the Lord to put your mind at ease, to put your body in total relaxation at bedtime, and to rest peacefully. **It's a simple prayer.**

"Ask and ye shall receive." The well-known Bible verse carries a lot of weight. Please don't knock it, if you haven't tried it. *Sleep Great for Life* works. The process defined in this book works even more quickly when you rely on this final step.

Not everyone is religious, but that doesn't mean you can't tap into the power of the world's most widely read, widely published, and well known book. The Bible is full of verses that can help put your mind at ease. I present just a few of the many verses found in the Bible that relate to the promise. All of life's great problems are addressed in The Book. The Bible offers the following great promises:

"Peace I leave you, my peace I give unto you. . . . Let not your heart be troubled, neither let it be afraid." – John 14:27

"Cast all your anxiety onto Him because He cares for you." – 1 Peter 5:7

"I am with you and will watch over you wherever you go." – Genesis 28:15

"The Lord is good, a refuge in times of trouble. He cares for those who trust in him." – Nahum 1:7

"The Lord is the strength of my Life. In this I will have confidence." – Psalms 27:1

"But those who trust in the Lord will find new strength. They will soar high on wings like eagles. They will run and not grow weary. They will walk and not faint." – Isaiah 40:31

"Fret not thyself." – Psalm 37:1

"Don't worry about anything; instead, pray about everything. Tell God what you need, and thank him for all he has done." – Philippians 4:6

"I can do all things through Christ which strengthen me." – Philippians 4:13

"Let us think of ways to motivate one another to acts of love and good works." – Hebrews 10:24

"If God be for us, who can be against us?" – Romans 8:31

"The Kingdom of God is within you." – Luke 17:21

"Be still and know that I am God." – Psalm 46:10

"This is the day the Lord has made. I will rejoice and be glad in it." – Psalm 118:24

Give these verses a try. Take one for each day of the week and repeat several times throughout the day. Do this every day for two consecutive weeks, as there are 14 verses presented here. That last one (Psalm 118:24) is an especially great verse to start every day with. Psalm 46:10 is also a great verse to repeat when you first lie down to bed in order to put yourself into a peaceful frame of mind.

Make sure to repeat the verse of the day as you lie in bed ready for the night. Remember, "Ask and you will receive." Besides, what do you have to lose? Why not draw from the higher power that is God? He is there to help you. You just have to ask.

RESOURCES

Sleep-Related Websites

www.sleepeducation.com – wealth of resources from the American Academy of Sleep Medicine

www.sleepfoundation.org – tools from the National Sleep Foundation

www.twitter.com/sleepgreat – social networking site for this book

www.sleepgreatforlife.com – the blog for this book which publishes weekly articles on the subject

www.stanford.edu/~dement – The Sleep Well from Dr. William Dement of Stanford University

REFERENCES

Chapter 1

1. Quoted in Dash, J. (December 23, 2007). "How to sleep better." *Parade*.

2. Mishori, R. (June 7, 2009). "Stay healthy." *Parade*.

3. ANI. (September 6, 2009). "Lack of sleep may lead to cardiac problems." Retreived from http://articles.timesofindia.indiatimes.com/2009-09-06/health/28060958_1_blood-pressure-insomniacs-sleepers

4. "Lack of sleep makes life difficult." (July 4, 2007). Medical-Health-Care-Information.com

5. United States Department of Health and Human Services. 2007.

6. The National Sleep Foundation. (2002). *2002 "Sleep in America" poll*. Retrieved from: http://www.sleepfoundation.org/article/sleep-america-polls/2002-adult-sleep-habits

7. *Consumer Reports*. (September 2008).

8. Shellenbarger, S. "Sleep-deprived nation." *Wall Street Journal*.

9. Wikipedia.com. Author unknown.

10. "Many sleep best when they sleep alone." (March 11, 2007). *New York Times.*

Chapter 2

1. Lena D. Edwards, MD., "Stop Stress Before It Stops You." http://chrisrosenthaldesign.com/sp/?p=2347

Chapter 4

1. "Stress and obesity." (October 15, 2009). *The Courier Journal.*

2. Rowley, L. (June 4, 2009). "Be careful what you wish for." Retreived from:

   http://finance.yahoo.com/expert/article/moneyhappy/167884

Chapter 5

1. O'Connor, A. (September 21, 2009). "The claim: Lack of sleep increases the risk of catching a cold." www.nytimes.com/2009/09/22/health/22real.html?ref=anahadoconnor.

2. *Health And Wellness for Life Remedy.* (Fall 2009).

Chapter 6

1. Rosenfeld, Dr. Isadore. "Doctor of the Heart: My Life in Medicine." Reported on FOX News.

Chapter 7

1. Kase, L. M. (October 2007). "The magic power of sleep." *Readers Digest.*

ABOUT THE AUTHOR

Rich Nilsen is the founder and President of All Star Press, an independent book publisher. He has written for several different, professional trade publications over the past two decades and, in addition to this book, is the author of *The Road to Recovery: Overcoming and Moving Beyond Your Grief.*

To learn more about All Star Press and Rich Nilsen's other publications, or just want to follow the latest news about e-books or e-readers, please visit www.allstarpress.com.

You can visit the Blog for "Sleep Great for Life" at www.sleepgreatforlife.com

FEEDBACK

Please let me know if *Sleep Great for Life* has the type of impact in your life that I fully expect it to have. My goal in writing this book is that many lives will be transformed with rejuvenating and energizing great sleep.

If this book has impacted your life, please take a few seconds and shoot me a note at allstarpress@verizon.net.

POST A REVIEW

If this book helped you, then please consider spreading the word. You can take a few minutes to write a positive review on the site where you purchased this book.

If you have a blog, you could write a short book review on your site.

For those of you with Facebook, Twitter, or other social-networking accounts, feel free to share information about this book with your friends and fans.

Thank you for your purchase of *Sleep Great for Life*.

Thank you and God bless.

AllStar
PRESS

ALL STAR PRESS
PUBLICATIONS & WEBSITES:

The Eye Floaters Solution by Chantal Romy

The House that Richard Built by James D. Smith

Quiet Spaces: Hearing God's Call in a Noisy World
By James Hale

The Road to Recovery: Overcoming & Moving Beyond Your
Grief
By Rich Nilsen

COMING SOON! *My Wild Ride* by Susan Bump

Monica Loves the Movies by Stephen Wolfson

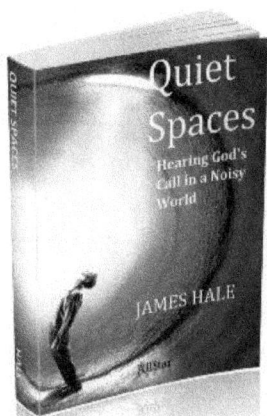

DO YOU WANT MORE OUT OF YOUR WORK?

WOULD YOU LIKE TO LEARN WHAT YOUR TRUE CALLING IS?

QUIET SPACES: Hearing God's Call in a Noisy World

By James Hale

Learn to hear God's calling in your life and apply it successfully to your day job. This book includes a 45-day devotional.

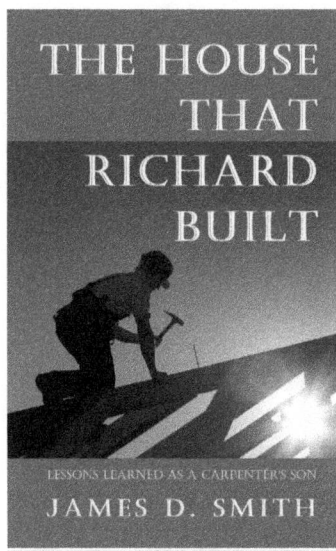

THE HOUSE THAT RICHARD BUILT:
Life Lessons as a Carpenter's Son
By James D. Smith
Rated 4.5 Stars on Amazon.com

This is a powerful book from Kentucky Pastor James D. Smith that details the life lessons he learned as the son of a carpenter. It is currently available exclusively through Amazon.com for the Kindle eReader, Kindle App, and online through the Kindle Cloud.

It's true that we are all carpenters; we are all building something. We are building families, marriages, careers, relationships, and legacies. Do we have the right type of tools and instruction to build the life we want? You can learn about these power tools for life in the new e-book "The House that Richard Built."

Order it today on Amazon.com or at AllStarPress.com

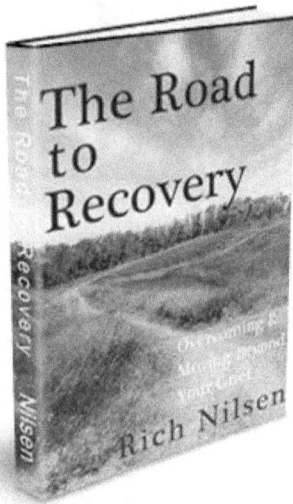

Rated 5 Stars on Amazon.com

Help is here if you are suffering the loss of a loved one. As helpful as friends and family can be, often times they can not provide the understanding you need because they don't know what you are going through. Rich Nilsen lost his college sweetheart and wife of four and a half years in a commercial airline crash in 1997. She was only 27 years old.

In "The Road to Recovery" Nilsen discusses that you come to a crossroads in your life when you lose someone very dear to you. To help you choose the right path, it is vital to read the work of someone who knows full well the deep sorrow you feel and can provide both comfort and practical advice that works. That is where this book comes in.

Testimonials

"The contents are amazing and profound. Your words rang loud and true when I read them. Wish I had found this book earlier." - Terry Welch, sister to Michael Ryan lost on Comair flight 5196, Aug. 27, 2006.

"I just read The Road to Recovery. It was so informative. I am founder and director of a bereavement support group for parents who have lost a child." - Ann Carruci, HANDS (Healing and Nurturing Distraught Survivors)

"We would love to get a copy of The Road to Recovery and see if we can incorporate it into our resource materials in some way. Again, I want to thank you for developing this material and for your incredible effort to reach out to those suffering from the 9/11 disaster." - April Naturale, New York State Director, Project Liberty.

"Be assured that we will have your support guides distributed to those who have lost a loved one in the tragedy of Sept. 11th. Thank you for all you have done to help alleviate some of the pain borne by loved ones of those who died on September 11th [2001]." - Rev. Msgr. Gregory Mustaciuolo, the Secretary to His Eminence, Edward Cardinal Egan.

"This book contains so many insightful, appropriate and helpful ideas and suggestions. God bless you." - Kelly Markillie, pastoral counselor at The Cathedral of Christ The King, Atlanta, GA.

"I lost my son in the World Trade Center [911] and I found your book so comforting." - Patricia Noah, mother of Leonard M. Castrianno, Cantor Fitzgerald, 105th floor World Trade Center.

"The Road to Recovery" is jam packed with helpful advice and resources to guide through this turbulent time, and make sure you get on the road to a better life. Healing is around the corner.

If you or someone you love is dealing with sorrow, this book will be of great comfort and offer invaluable bereavement advice that you can begin to apply today. Each day can and will get easier. Download this book to your eReader or PC today.

http://www.griefhelp.org
http://twitter.com/griefhelp

ALLSTARPRESS.COM - Books That Change Lives

Publications, both print and ebook, from All Star Press are also available online through all major online retailers.

NOTES

_____

_____

_____

_____

_____

_____

_____

_____

_____

_____

_____

_____

_____

_____

_____

_____

_____

_____

_____

_____

_____

_____

_____

_____

_____

_____

_____

_____

_____

_____

_____

_____

_____

_____

_____

_____

_____

_____

_____

_____

_____

_____

_____

_____

_____

_____

_____

_____

_____

_____

_____

_____

_____

_____

_____

_____

_____

_____

_____

_____

_____

_____

_____

_____

_____

_____

_____

_____

_____

_____

_____

_____

_____

_____

_____

_____

_____

_____

_____

_____

_____

_____

_____

_____

_____

_____

_____

_____

_____

_____

_____

_____

_____

_____

_____

_____

_____

_____

_____

_____

_____

_____

_____

_____

_____

_____

_____

_____

_____

_____

_____

_____

_____

_____

_____

_____

_____

_____

_____

_____

_____

_____

_____

_____

_____

AllStar

P R E S S

www.allstarpress.com

.

www.ingramcontent.com/pod-product-compliance
Lightning Source LLC
Chambersburg PA
CBHW030024290326
41934CB00005B/471